ESSENTIAL VITAMIN NUTRITION

What Your Body Really Needs

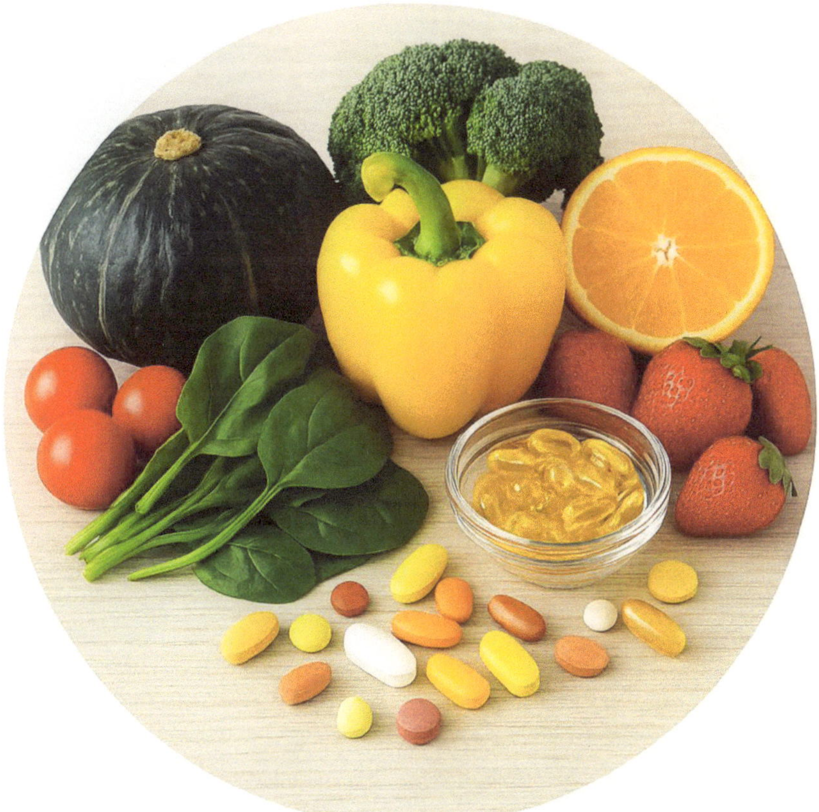

Our Collections

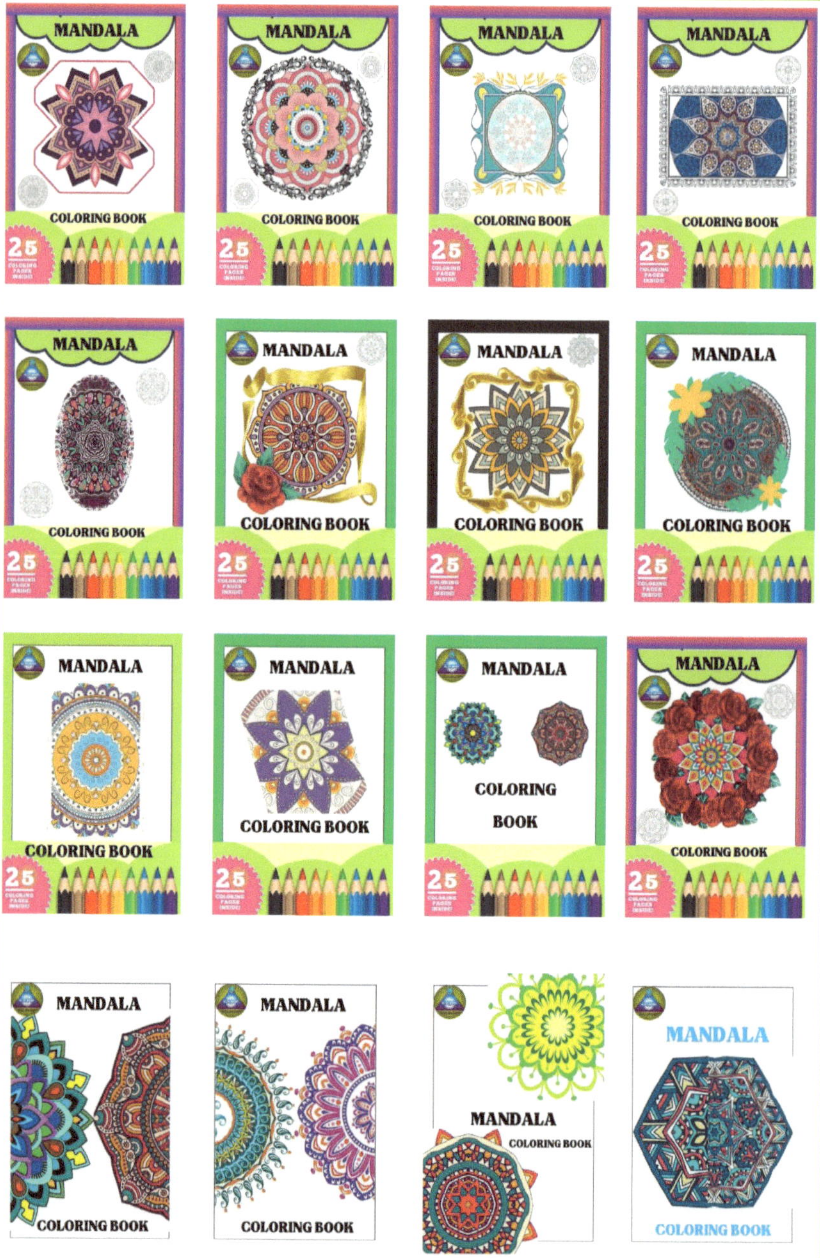

PUBLISHED BY THE BLJ KTS SERVICES

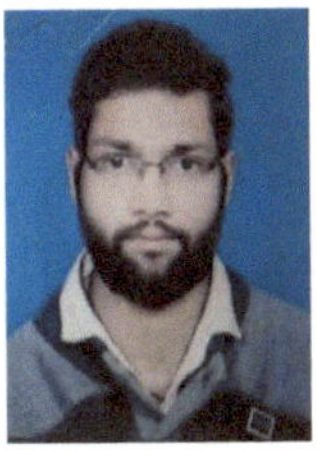

Disclaimer

Author: ***Mayank Goel.***

Printed By: ***Geniux Technologies, Bilari, Moradabad, U.P., INDIA***

ISBN No: 978-81-995902-3-6

Terms and Conditions

LEGAL NOTICE

The Publisher has made every effort to ensure that the information contained in this book is accurate and complete at the time of publication. However, due to the rapidly changing nature of the Internet and related fields, the Publisher makes no representations or warranties regarding the accuracy, applicability, fitness, or completeness of the contents.

While all attempts have been made to verify the information provided, the Publisher assumes no responsibility for errors, omissions, or interpretations of the subject matter. Any perceived slights of individuals, groups, or organizations are unintentional.

This book does not guarantee any results, earnings, or outcomes. Readers are encouraged to use their own judgment and consider their personal circumstances when making decisions.

This publication is not intended to serve as legal, financial, accounting, or business advice. Readers are strongly advised to consult qualified professionals in these fields for specific guidance.

Table Of Contents

Foreword

In today's fast-paced world, many people rely on vitamins to supply the essential nutrients their bodies need to function at their best. This growing dependence often stems from busy lifestyles that leave little time for preparing well-balanced meals. In addition, many modern food choices fail to provide the complete range of vitamins required for optimal health.

This guide provides the essential information you need to understand vitamins and how they support your overall well-being.

Essential Vitamin Nutrition: What Your Body Really Needs

Chapter 1:

The Importance of Vitamins in Human Nutrition

Synopsis

Vitamins are essential nutrients that play a crucial role in keeping the body functioning at its best. They help release energy from the foods we eat and support vital processes such as maintaining healthy skin, strengthening the nervous system, and renewing red blood cells.

Without adequate vitamins, the body cannot sustain the continuous repair, growth, and vitality needed for overall health.

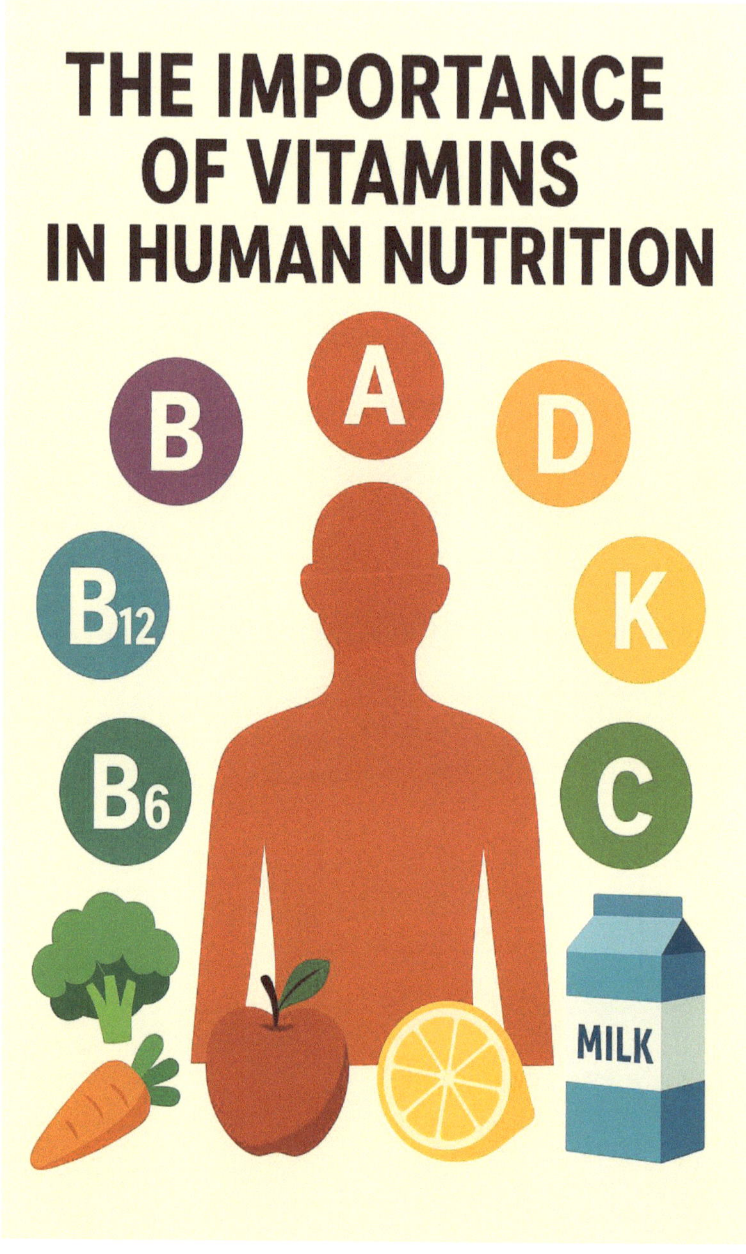
THE IMPORTANCE
OF VITAMINS
IN HUMAN NUTRITION
B
A
D
B12
K
B6
C
MILK

The Basics

Vitamins are generally divided into two main categories: **fat-soluble vitamins** and **water-soluble vitamins**, each playing distinct roles in maintaining health.

Fat-soluble vitamins include **A, D, E, and K**. These vitamins dissolve in fat, can be stored in the body, and are found in foods such as **vegetable oils, nuts, seeds, egg yolks, fish oils, whole grains,** and **dark leafy greens**. Because the body stores these vitamins, excess intake—especially through supplements—can lead to toxicity.

Water-soluble vitamins include **vitamin C** and the **B-vitamin family** (thiamin, riboflavin, niacin, folate, biotin, and pantothenic acid). These vitamins help the body produce energy, support the nervous system, maintain healthy skin, and aid cell regeneration. Since the body does not store water-soluble vitamins in large amounts, they must be replenished regularly through diet.

Modern Considerations for Today's Lifestyle

In today's world, several factors influence how our bodies absorb and use vitamins:

1. **Busy lifestyles and processed foods**
Many people rely on packaged or fast foods, which often lack essential nutrients. Even when food is fortified, it may not provide the full spectrum of vitamins needed for optimal health.

2. **Declining nutrient quality in food**
Modern farming practices, soil depletion, and long storage times can reduce the vitamin content of fruits and vegetables, making it harder to meet daily requirements from diet alone.

3. **Increased indoor lifestyles**
More time spent indoors has led to widespread **vitamin D deficiency**, as sunlight exposure is the primary natural source of this vitamin.

4. **Special diets and restrictions**
Vegan, vegetarian, keto, and gluten-free diets can unintentionally

create gaps in certain vitamins such as B12, iron, and folate, making supplementation more common.

5. Stress and environmental factors
Chronic stress, pollution, and poor sleep can increase the body's demand for vitamins—especially C and B complex vitamins—which are essential for immune function and stress regulation.

Supplement Use Today

Multivitamins and targeted supplements can help fill nutritional gaps, but they must be used wisely. Some vitamins do not interact well together, and fat-soluble vitamins can accumulate in the body, potentially causing toxicity. Interactions with medications—such as blood thinners, antibiotics, or thyroid treatments—can also pose risks.

Because of this, modern health experts recommend **personalized supplementation**, ideally based on dietary habits, medical conditions, and individual needs rather than one-size-fits-all solutions.

Chapter 2:

The Dangers of Vitamin Deficiency

Synopsis

Vitamin consumption still falls short of ideal levels for many people around the world. Meeting the body's daily nutritional requirements is becoming increasingly difficult due to several modern factors.

These include the rising cost of supplements, inconsistent or poorly planned diets, limited intake of nutritious foods, and reduced access to fresh fruits and vegetables. Additionally, the widespread preference for processed, fast, and convenience foods further contributes to inadequate vitamin intake.

Even in regions where supplements are widely available, many individuals do not use them correctly or consistently. Busy schedules, misinformation about nutrition, and the growing trend of restrictive diets can make maintaining balanced vitamin levels more challenging than ever.

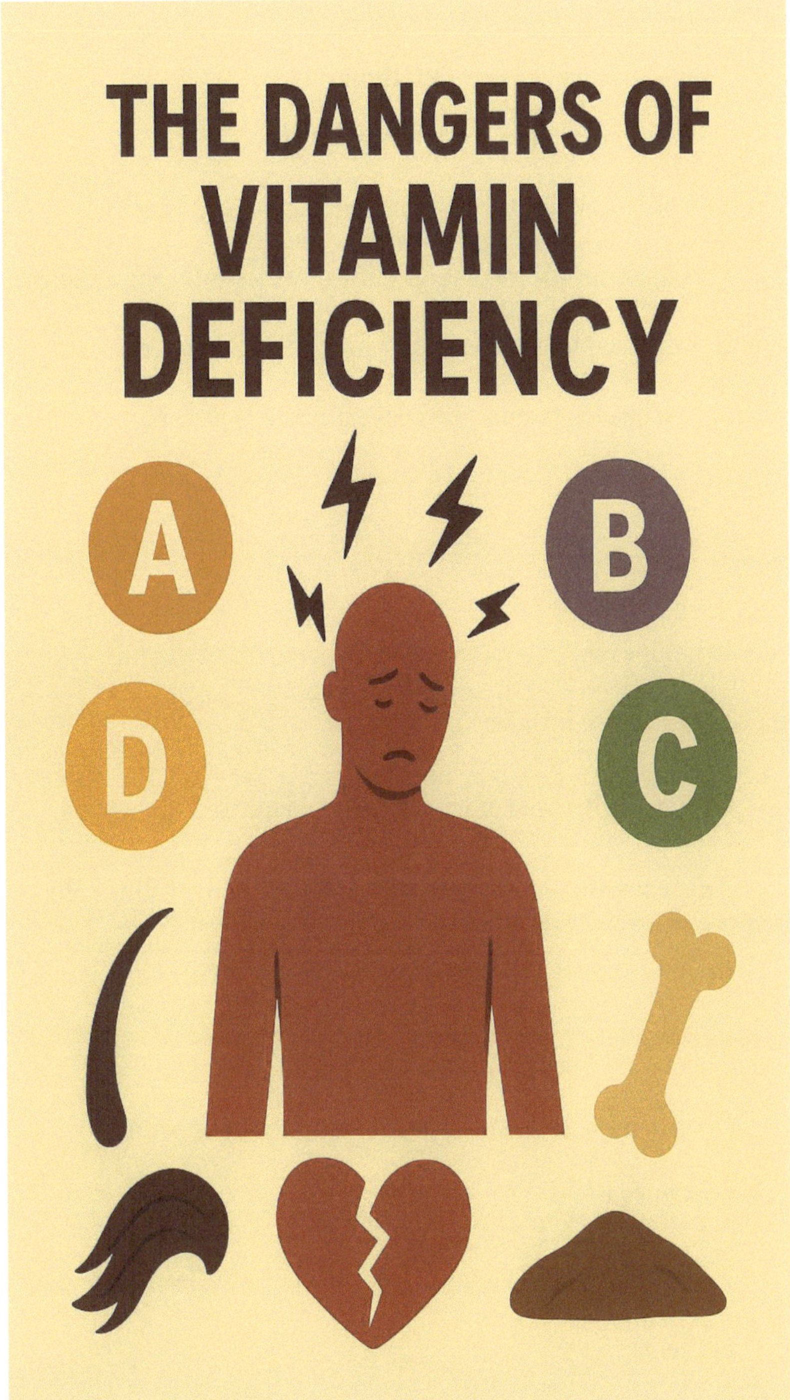
THE DANGERS OF
VITAMIN
DEFICIENCY
A
B
D
C

The Risks

Vitamin deficiencies place the body at higher risk for various illnesses and can lead to suboptimal physical and mental performance. Common signs include low energy, difficulty concentrating, frequent fatigue, weakened immunity, poor skin health, and slow healing. Without adequate vitamins, the body struggles to perform daily tasks efficiently and loses the ability to repair itself properly.

Certain groups remain at significantly higher risk for vitamin deficiencies. These include:

- **Older adults**, who often have reduced nutrient absorption
- **Adolescents**, due to rapid growth and irregular eating habits
- **Pregnant and breastfeeding women**, whose nutrient needs increase
- **People who consume excessive alcohol or smoke cigarettes**
- **Vegetarians and vegans**, who may lack B12, iron, and other nutrients

- **Individuals on restrictive diets or fasting programs**
- **People with chronic illnesses**, particularly gastrointestinal disorders
- **Users of certain medications**, such as contraceptives, laxatives, and long-term prescriptions
- **Individuals with sedentary routines or extremely hectic lifestyles**

In today's world, additional factors such as chronic stress, poor sleep, excessive screen time, and limited outdoor exposure (leading to widespread vitamin D deficiency) have further intensified these risks.

Examples of Common Deficiencies

- **Vitamin A deficiency**
  Continues to be a leading cause of preventable blindness in children worldwide and increases vulnerability to infections.
- **Vitamin D deficiency**
  Extremely common today due to indoor lifestyles. It contributes to brittle bones, weak immunity, depression, and chronic fatigue.

- **Vitamin E deficiency**

  Affects brain function, immune strength, and cardiovascular health. While rare, it is increasing among individuals with fat absorption issues.

- **Vitamin B deficiencies** (B12, B6, folate)

  Can cause severe fatigue, nerve problems, anemia, mood disturbances, and cognitive decline. These deficiencies are especially common among older adults, vegetarians, and people under chronic stress.

Chapter 3:
Kinds Of Vitamins

Synopsis

Vitamins are essential nutrients that the body needs in small but consistent amounts to function properly. They are divided into two main categories based on how they are absorbed, stored, and used within the body: **fat-soluble vitamins** and **water-soluble vitamins**. Each group plays a distinct role in supporting overall health, growth, and daily body functions.

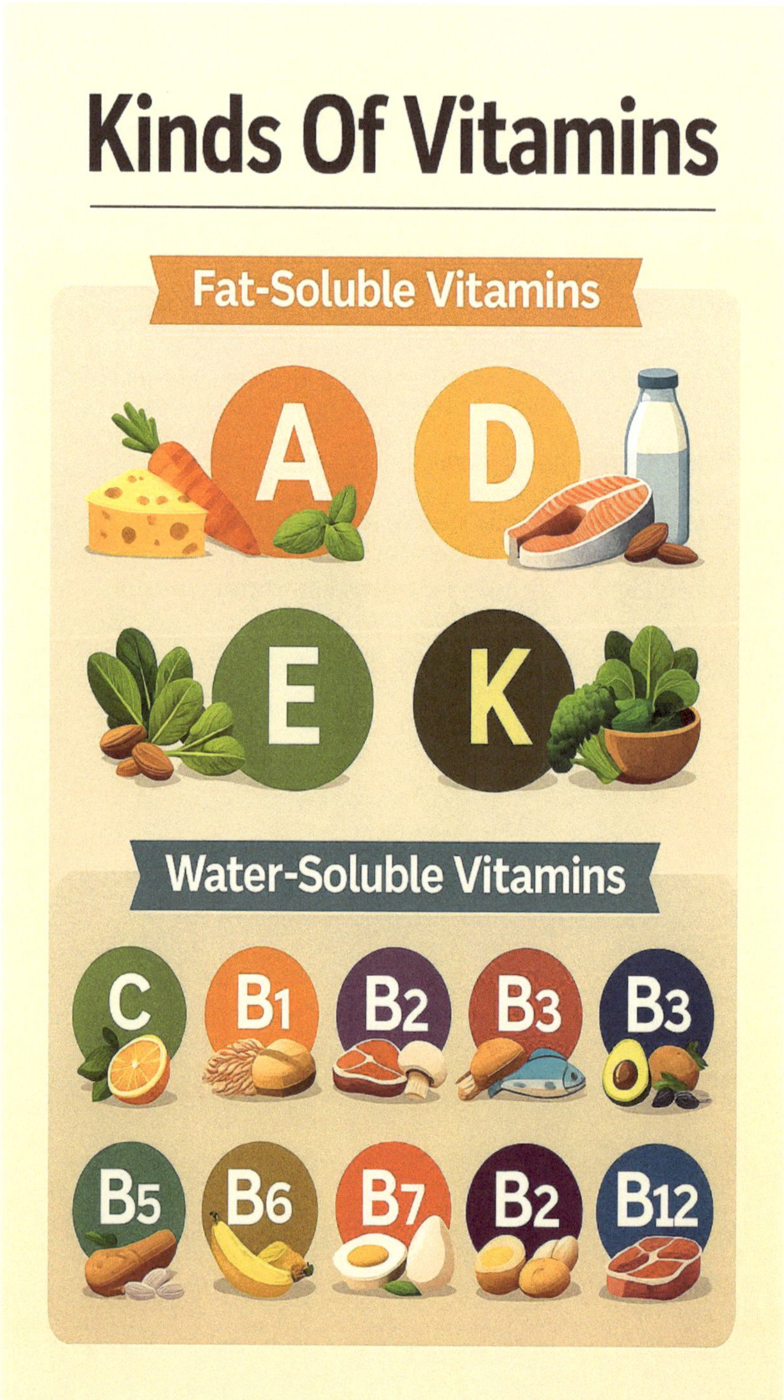
Kinds Of Vitamins
Fat-Soluble Vitamins
A
D
E
K
Water-Soluble Vitamins
C
B1
B2
B3
B3
B5
B6
B7
B2
B12

1. Fat-Soluble Vitamins

These vitamins dissolve in fat and can be stored in the body's fatty tissues and liver. Because of this, they do not need to be consumed daily, but excessive intake can lead to toxicity.

The fat-soluble vitamins include:

- **Vitamin A**

  Supports vision, immune function, and healthy skin.

- **Vitamin D**

  Essential for bone health, calcium absorption, immunity, and mood regulation. Modern indoor lifestyles have made vitamin D deficiency extremely common.

- **Vitamin E**

  Acts as a powerful antioxidant, protecting cells from damage and supporting brain and heart health.

- **Vitamin K**

  Important for blood clotting and bone metabolism.

Sources: nuts, seeds, fish oils, egg yolks, dairy fat, leafy greens, and fortified foods.

2. Water-Soluble Vitamins

These vitamins dissolve in water and are not stored in large amounts by the body. Because excess amounts are excreted through urine, they must be replenished daily through food or supplementation.

The water-soluble vitamins include:

Vitamin C

Strengthens the immune system, supports skin and tissue repair, enhances iron absorption, and functions as an antioxidant.

B-Complex Vitamins

A group of eight essential vitamins that work together to support metabolism, brain function, energy production, and nerve health:

- **B1 (Thiamin)** – Helps convert food into energy.
- **B2 (Riboflavin)** – Important for cell function and energy metabolism.
- **B3 (Niacin)** – Supports nervous system and digestive health.

- **B5 (Pantothenic Acid)** – Necessary for hormone and energy production.
- **B6 (Pyridoxine)** – Supports brain development and immune function.
- **B7 (Biotin)** – Essential for healthy hair, skin, and nails.
- **B9 (Folate/Folic Acid)** – Crucial for DNA formation and pregnancy health.
- **B12 (Cobalamin)** – Needed for red blood cell formation and neurological function.

Sources: citrus fruits, berries, leafy greens, whole grains, beans, nuts, dairy products, meat, eggs, and fortified foods.

Today's Nutrition Challenge

Despite the variety of vitamins available in everyday foods, many people still struggle to meet their daily needs due to fast-paced lifestyles, processed diets, poor food quality, and limited access to fresh produce. Understanding the kinds of vitamins and where they come from is the first step toward maintaining a balanced and healthy nutritional profile.

Chapter 4:

Food Sources of Essential Vitamins

Synopsis

A balanced diet remains the most natural and effective way to supply the body with the vitamins it needs. Different foods provide different nutrients, and understanding where vitamins come from helps you make healthier choices every day. Below is a clear guide to the best food sources of essential vitamins, based on current nutritional knowledge and today's common dietary patterns.

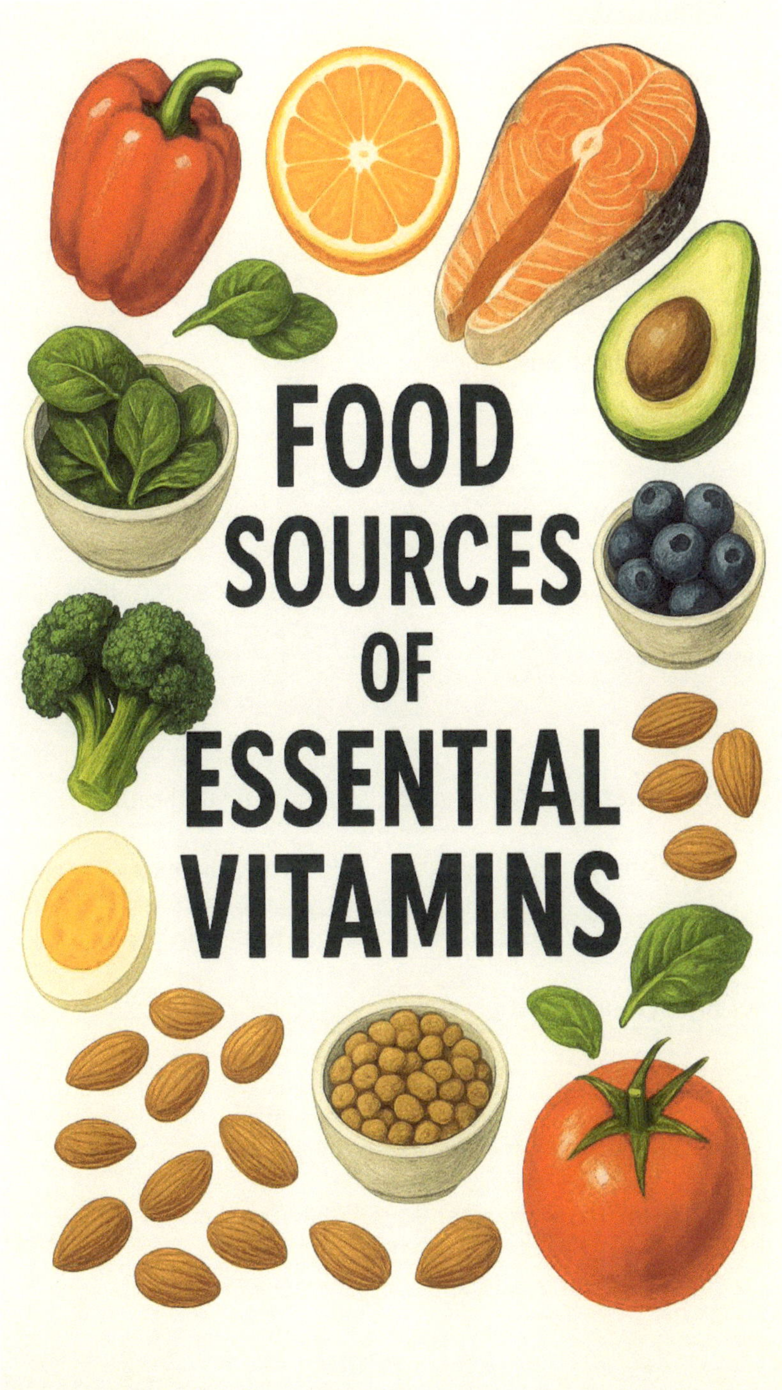
FOOD
SOURCES
OF
ESSENTIAL
VITAMINS

1. Vitamin A

Benefits: Vision, immunity, skin health

Sources:

- Carrots, sweet potatoes, pumpkins
- Spinach, kale, and other leafy greens
- Liver and fish oils
- Eggs and fortified dairy products

---

2. Vitamin B-Complex

Benefits: Energy production, brain function, red blood cell formation

Sources:

- **B1 (Thiamin):** Whole grains, sunflower seeds, beans
- **B2 (Riboflavin):** Eggs, dairy, lean meats, almonds
- **B3 (Niacin):** Chicken, tuna, peanuts, brown rice
- **B5 (Pantothenic Acid):** Avocados, broccoli, yogurt, mushrooms
- **B6 (Pyridoxine):** Bananas, chickpeas, salmon, potatoes
- **B7 (Biotin):** Eggs, nuts, seeds, sweet potatoes
- **B9 (Folate):** Lentils, spinach, asparagus, citrus fruits

- **B12 (Cobalamin):** Meat, fish, dairy, fortified plant milks (important for vegans)

---

3. Vitamin C

Benefits: Immunity, collagen production, antioxidant protection

Sources:

- Oranges, lemons, limes
- Strawberries, kiwis, pineapples
- Bell peppers, tomatoes, broccoli

---

4. Vitamin D

Benefits: Bone health, immunity, mood regulation

Sources:

- Sunlight (primary natural source)
- Fatty fish (salmon, tuna, mackerel)
- Egg yolks
- Fortified milk, cereals, and plant-based beverages

Note: Many people today are vitamin D deficient due to indoor lifestyles, making sunlight and fortified foods especially important.

---

5. Vitamin E

Benefits: Antioxidant support, heart health, skin protection

Sources:

- Almonds, sunflower seeds, hazelnuts
- Spinach, Swiss chard
- Vegetable oils (sunflower, safflower, olive)

---

6. Vitamin K

Benefits: Blood clotting, bone health

Sources:

- Kale, spinach, broccoli, Brussels sprouts
- Green beans
- Fermented foods (such as natto)

Modern Note

Due to busy lifestyles, processed foods, and reduced nutrient quality in modern produce, many individuals still fail to get sufficient vitamin levels even with a varied diet. Incorporating whole foods, fresh produce, and fortified items can help close nutritional gaps, while supplements can be used when dietary sources are limited.

Chapter 5:

How to Select the Best Vitamins for Your Health

Synopsis

Choosing the right vitamins has become increasingly important in today's world, where busy schedules, processed foods, and environmental factors can make it difficult to meet daily nutritional needs. With so many supplements on the market, selecting the best vitamins can feel overwhelming. However, understanding your body's requirements and recognizing the quality of available products can help you make informed and health-supportive decisions.

1. Understand Your Personal Needs

Every individual has different nutritional requirements. Factors that influence your vitamin needs include:

- **Age** – Children, adults, and seniors require different vitamin levels.
- **Gender** – Women may need more iron or folate; men may need more B vitamins.

- **Life stage** – Pregnancy, breastfeeding, and aging change nutritional demands.
- **Diet** – Vegetarians, vegans, and those on keto or low-carb diets may lack certain vitamins.
- **Health conditions** – Digestive issues, chronic illnesses, or medications can affect nutrient absorption.
- **Lifestyle** – Stress, lack of sleep, and minimal sunlight exposure (affecting vitamin D) can increase vitamin needs.

Before selecting vitamins, identify what your body may be lacking.

---

2. Focus on Food First

Supplements should support—not replace—a healthy diet. Always aim to get vitamins from natural food sources such as fruits, vegetables, whole grains, nuts, seeds, legumes, and lean protein. Foods contain additional beneficial compounds like fiber, antioxidants, and phytonutrients that supplements cannot fully replicate.

Use supplements only to fill the gaps that diet alone cannot cover.

HOW TO SELECT THE BEST VITAMINS FOR YOUR HEALTH

Start With Your Actual Needs

Not everyone needs every vitamin. Begin by reviewing:

- Your diet
- Your lifestyle
- Your health concerns
- Symptoms like firedness, hair fail, low immunity, muscramps

Tip: Adoctor or dietician can help identify deficiencies through a simple blood test (Vitamin B12, D3, Iron, Folate, ete:)

Choose Vitamins Based on Purpose

Energy & Tiredness
Vitamin B12, B-Complex, Iron

Immunity
Vitamin C, Vitamin D3, Zinc

Bone & Muscle Health
Vitamin D3 + K2, Calcium Magnesium

Sicn, Hair & Nails
Biotin, Vitamin E, Omega-3, Collager

Heart Health
Omega-3, CoQ10, Vitamin K2

Eye Health
Vitamin A, Lutein, Zeaxanthin

Pick the Right Form

Look for vitamins are one absorbed better than others.

- Vitamin D3 (better than D2)
- Methylcobalamin B12 (better than eyanocobalamin)
- Chelated minerals like magnesium glycinate or zinc picolinate
- Omega-3 (EPA/DHA) from fish oil or algae oil

Summary: Best Vitamins Are...

✔ Based on your health needs

Avoid Mega-Doses

More is NOT better. Avold supplements that give more than 100–200% of your daily requirements

unless prescribed

Prefer Food First

Whole foods provide fiber, antioxidants phytonutrients that no tablet can replace

Supplements should fill. gaps, not replace your diet

3. Choose High-Quality Supplements

Not all vitamins are created equal. When selecting supplements, look for products that meet these quality standards:

- **Third-party testing** (NSF, USP, Informed-Choice)
- **No unnecessary additives** or artificial fillers
- **Clear labeling** of ingredient amounts and forms
- **Bioavailable forms** (e.g., methylated B vitamins, D3 instead of D2)
- **Reputable brands** with transparent manufacturing practices

Avoid supplements with vague labels or extremely high doses that exceed recommended daily values.

---

4. Understand Vitamin Forms and Absorption

Different forms of vitamins absorb differently in the body. Some key points:

- **Vitamin D3** is better absorbed than D2.
- **Methylcobalamin (B12)** is more bioavailable than cyanocobalamin.

- **Natural vitamin E** (d-alpha-tocopherol) is more effective than synthetic forms.
- **Calcium citrate** absorbs better than calcium carbonate for people with low stomach acid.

Choosing the right form can significantly improve how well your body uses the vitamin.

---

5. Consider Your Current Health Conditions and Medications

Certain vitamins interact with medications or medical conditions. For example:

- Vitamin K can interfere with blood thinners.
- High-dose vitamin A may be harmful during pregnancy.
- Calcium and iron can affect the absorption of thyroid medication.
- Some supplements may overstimulate individuals with anxiety disorders.

Consulting a healthcare professional is especially important if you take prescription medication.

---

6. Avoid Mega doses Unless Prescribed

More is not always better. Some vitamins—especially fat-soluble ones like **A, D, E, and K**—can accumulate in the body and become toxic over time. Even water-soluble vitamins can cause adverse effects if taken in excessive amounts.

Aim for safe, balanced doses that meet daily requirements unless a doctor recommends otherwise.

---

7. Tailor Your Vitamins to Your Goals

People take vitamins for different reasons. You may select vitamins to support:

- **Energy and metabolism** – B complex, iron
- **Immune health** – vitamins C, D, zinc
- **Bone strength** – calcium, magnesium, vitamin D, vitamin K2
- **Brain health** – omega-3s, vitamin E, B12
- **Skin and hair health** – biotin, collagen, vitamin A

Choosing supplements that align with your specific health goals leads to better results.

---

8. Reevaluate Regularly

Your vitamin needs may change over time due to age, diet, routines, health status, or life stages. Reviewing your supplements every few months—preferably with guidance from a doctor or nutritionist—ensures you're getting what your body currently needs.

Chapter 6:

Essential Vitamins for Infants

Synopsis

Infants grow and develop at an extraordinary pace, making proper nutrition crucial during the earliest stages of life. While breast milk or formula is generally designed to provide most of the nutrients a baby needs, certain vitamins play especially important roles in supporting healthy growth, immunity, brain development, and bone strength. Understanding these essential vitamins helps parents ensure their baby receives a strong foundation for lifelong health.

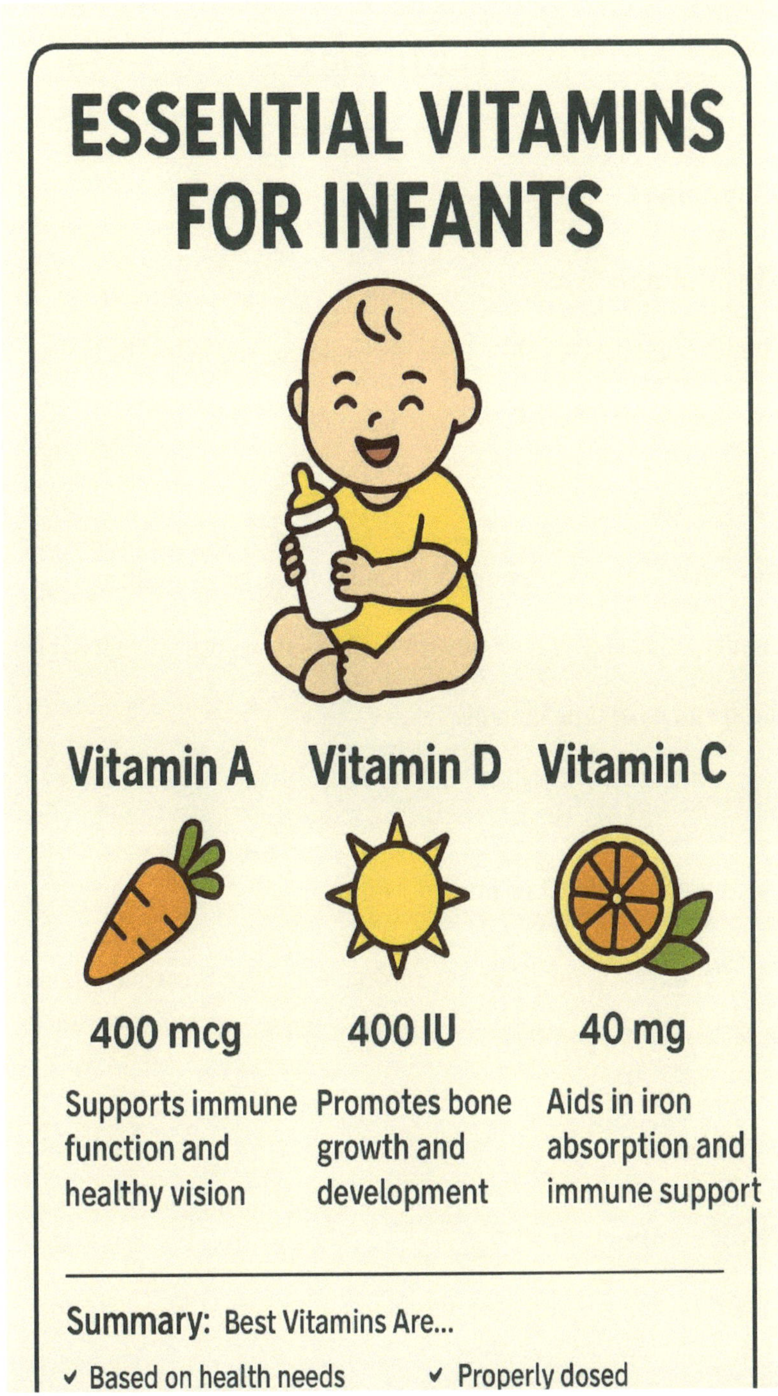
ESSENTIAL VITAMINS FOR INFANTS
Vitamin A
Vitamin D
Vitamin C
400 mcg
400 IU
40 mg
Supports immune function and healthy vision
Promotes bone growth and development
Aids in iron absorption and immune support
Summary: Best Vitamins Are...
✔ Based on health needs
✔ Properly dosed

For Infants

1. Vitamin D

Why it's important:

Vitamin D supports healthy bone development and helps the body absorb calcium. It also plays a role in immunity and overall growth.

Modern note:

Most infants do **not** get enough vitamin D from breast milk or sunlight, especially in regions with limited sun exposure or for babies who spend most time indoors.

Sources:

- Vitamin D–fortified infant formula
- Pediatric vitamin D drops (recommended for breastfed infants)

---

2. Vitamin A

Why it's important:

Supports vision development, immune system strength, and healthy skin.

Sources:

- Breast milk and formula
- Pureed orange and yellow vegetables (carrots, sweet potatoes) once solid foods begin

---

3. Vitamin C

Why it's important:

Strengthens the immune system, supports tissue repair, and aids iron absorption.

Sources (for babies eating solids):

- Mashed fruits such as oranges, strawberries, mangoes
- Vegetables like potatoes, broccoli, and tomatoes

Breast milk and formula naturally provide adequate vitamin C for infants under six months.

---

4. Vitamin B-Complex

Why it's important:

The B vitamins support brain development, energy production, healthy digestion, and the creation of new cells.

Key B vitamins for infants:

- **B2 (Riboflavin)** – growth of body tissues
- **B6** – brain and immune development
- **B9 (Folate)** – formation of red blood cells
- **B12** – essential for nerve and brain development

Sources:

- Breast milk and formula
- Pureed meats, eggs, fortified cereals (for older infants)

Note: Infants of vegan or vegetarian mothers may be at higher risk of B12 deficiency and may need pediatric guidance.

---

5. Vitamin E

Why it's important:

Acts as an antioxidant, protecting cells from damage and supporting healthy skin and eyes.

Sources:

- Breast milk and formula
- Small amounts in pureed vegetables and seeds (for older infants)

---

6. Vitamin K

Why it's important:

Helps blood clot properly and prevents dangerous internal bleeding.

Modern practice:

Infants are routinely given a **vitamin K injection at birth** to prevent deficiency, as breast milk contains very low levels.

Ensuring Infants Get the Right Vitamins

- **Breast milk or formula** should be the primary source of nutrition for the first 6 months.
- **Vitamin D supplementation** is recommended for most infants, especially if breastfed.
- As solid foods are introduced around 6 months, parents should offer a variety of nutrient-rich foods, including vegetables, fruits, whole grains, and soft meats.
- Always consult a pediatrician before giving any additional supplements to an infant.

Chapter 7:

Essential Vitamins for Adults

Synopsis

Adults rely on a wide range of vitamins to maintain energy, support immunity, promote mental clarity, and keep the body functioning at its best. As people age and life becomes busier, meeting daily vitamin requirements through diet alone can be challenging. Stress, processed foods, lack of sunlight, and lifestyle habits can all increase the risk of nutrient deficiencies. Understanding the essential vitamins for adults is key to maintaining long-term health and preventing chronic illness.

ESSENTIAL VITAMINS FOR ADULTS

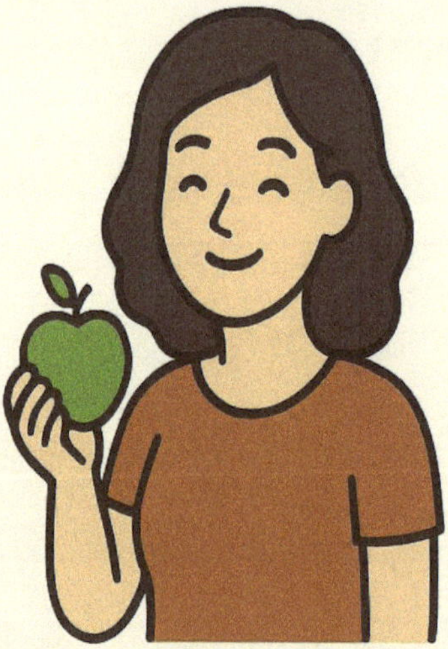

Vitamin A	Vitamin D	Vitamin C
	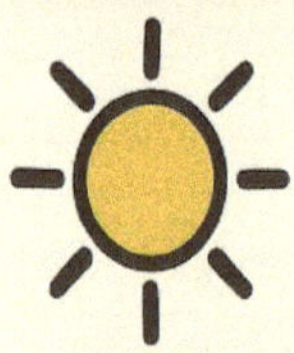	
900 mcg	20 mcg	90 mg
Vision and immune function	Bone and muscle health	Antioxidant and supports immune system

Summary: Best Vitamins Are...

- ✔ Based on health needs
- ✔ Properly dosed

For Grownups

1. Vitamin A

Why adults need it:

Supports vision, strengthens the immune system, keeps skin and mucous membranes healthy, and acts as an antioxidant.

Sources:

Carrots, spinach, kale, sweet potatoes, eggs, liver, fortified dairy products.

---

2. Vitamin B-Complex

The B vitamins work together to support metabolism, brain function, and energy production. They are especially important for adults who experience stress, fatigue, or have demanding schedules.

Key B vitamins for adults:

- **B1 (Thiamin):** Helps convert food into energy.
- **B2 (Riboflavin):** Supports cell growth and energy production.
- **B3 (Niacin):** Essential for nervous system and digestive health.

- **B5 (Pantothenic Acid):** Aids hormone production and metabolism.
- **B6 (Pyridoxine):** Supports brain function and healthy mood.
- **B7 (Biotin):** Promotes healthy skin, hair, and nails.
- **B9 (Folate):** Important for cell repair and healthy blood.
- **B12 (Cobalamin):** Essential for nerve function and red blood cell formation.

Sources:

Whole grains, eggs, dairy, meats, legumes, leafy greens, fortified cereals.

Note: Adults over 50, vegetarians, and vegans are at increased risk of B12 deficiency.

---

3. Vitamin C

Why adults need it:

Boosts immunity, repairs tissues, supports collagen formation, improves iron absorption, and functions as a powerful antioxidant.

Sources:

Citrus fruits, strawberries, kiwis, bell peppers, tomatoes, broccoli.

---

4. Vitamin D

Why adults need it:

Promotes bone health, supports immunity, improves mood, and may reduce inflammation.

Modern concern:

Due to indoor lifestyles, sunscreen use, and long work hours, vitamin D deficiency is widespread among adults.

Sources:

Sunlight, fortified milk, fatty fish (salmon, mackerel), egg yolks.

---

5. Vitamin E

Why adults need it:

Protects cells from oxidative damage, supports cardiovascular health, and boosts immune function.

Sources:

Nuts, seeds, vegetable oils, spinach, avocados.

---

6. Vitamin K

Why adults need it:

Plays a critical role in blood clotting and supports bone health, especially for aging adults.

Sources:

Kale, spinach, broccoli, Brussels sprouts, fermented foods.

---

7. Additional Vitamins of Special Importance

In today's lifestyle, certain vitamins may be especially important for adults:

- **Vitamin B12:** Essential for adults over 50, vegetarians, and anyone with digestive issues.
- **Vitamin D3 + K2:** A popular combination for bone and immune health.
- **Folate & B6 & B12:** Support heart health by regulating homocysteine levels.

Meeting Daily Needs

Adults can meet their vitamin requirements through a mix of:

- A varied diet rich in whole foods
- Adequate sunlight exposure (for vitamin D)
- Fortified foods when needed
- High-quality supplements (when recommended)

Stress, alcohol consumption, smoking, lack of sleep, and chronic illnesses can all increase the body's demand for certain vitamins. Regular health checkups and blood tests can help identify any deficiencies early.

Chapter 8:
Essential Vitamins for Senior

Synopsis

As people age, their bodies undergo significant changes that affect how vitamins are absorbed, stored, and utilized. Seniors often require higher levels of certain nutrients to maintain bone strength, cognitive health, immunity, and overall vitality. Factors such as reduced appetite, medical conditions, medication use, and decreased digestive efficiency make it increasingly important to ensure adequate vitamin intake during the senior years.

Understanding the essential vitamins for older adults can help prevent deficiencies, support independence, and improve quality of life.

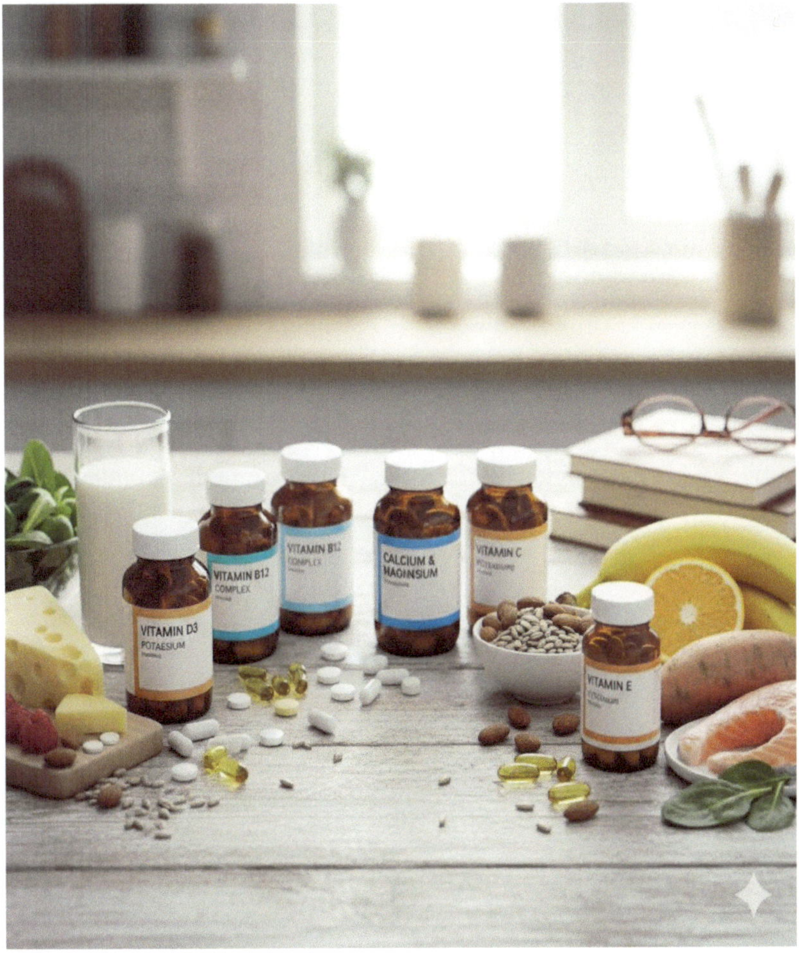

For Elders

1. Vitamin D

Why seniors need it:

Vitamin D plays a critical role in maintaining strong bones, muscle function, and immune health. It also helps reduce the risk of fractures and supports mood stability.

Modern concern:

Many seniors are deficient due to limited sunlight exposure, decreased skin synthesis, and digestive changes.

Sources:

Sunlight, fortified milk, fatty fish, egg yolks, vitamin D3 supplements.

---

2. Vitamin B12

Why seniors need it:

Vitamin B12 is essential for nerve health, red blood cell production, and cognitive function. Deficiency is strongly linked to memory loss, fatigue, and neuropathy.

Modern concern:

Older adults often have reduced stomach acid, making it harder to absorb B12 from food.

Sources:

Fish, poultry, eggs, dairy, fortified cereals, B12 supplements (often necessary for seniors).

---

3. Vitamin B6

Why seniors need it:

Supports brain function, helps regulate mood, and plays a role in immune system health.

Sources:

Bananas, poultry, whole grains, potatoes, nuts.

---

4. Vitamin C

Why seniors need it:

Boosts immunity, helps with wound healing, protects cells from damage, and enhances iron absorption.

Sources:

Citrus fruits, berries, tomatoes, peppers, broccoli.

---

5. Vitamin A

Why seniors need it:

Supports eye health, skin integrity, and immune function. However, seniors must be careful not to consume too much from supplements.

Sources:

Carrots, sweet potatoes, spinach, eggs, fortified dairy products.

---

6. Vitamin K2

Why seniors need it:

Vitamin K2 works with vitamin D to support bone strength and reduce the risk of fractures. It also supports cardiovascular health by helping regulate calcium placement in the body.

Sources:

Fermented foods (natto), cheese, eggs, leafy greens.

---

7. Vitamin E

Why seniors need it:

Acts as an antioxidant, supports immune function, and may help protect cognitive health.

Sources:

Nuts, seeds, spinach, avocados, vegetable oils.

Why Seniors Are at Higher Risk of Vitamin Deficiency

- Reduced appetite and smaller meals
- Difficulty chewing or swallowing certain foods
- Chronic illnesses affecting nutrient absorption
- Medications that interfere with vitamin metabolism
- Limited outdoor activity (affects vitamin D)
- Decreased stomach acid (affects B12, iron, calcium)

Ensuring Adequate Intake

To help seniors meet their nutritional needs:

- Include nutrient-rich foods in meals and snacks
- Choose fortified foods when necessary
- Consider high-quality senior-formulated multivitamins
- Get regular blood tests to monitor vitamin levels
- Consult healthcare providers before starting supplements

A balanced approach can help maintain energy levels, protect bone and brain health, and support a healthy immune system during the senior years.

Chapter 9:

<u>How to Prevent Vitamin Overdose</u>

Synopsis

While vitamins are essential for maintaining good health, taking them in excessive amounts can be harmful. Vitamin overdose—also known as **hypervitaminosis**—usually occurs when people take more supplements than their body needs, especially fat-soluble vitamins that can build up in the body over time. With the increasing popularity of high-dose supplements, energy boosters, and "mega" multivitamins, understanding how to prevent vitamin overdose is more important than ever.

Here are effective ways to ensure safe and balanced vitamin intake.

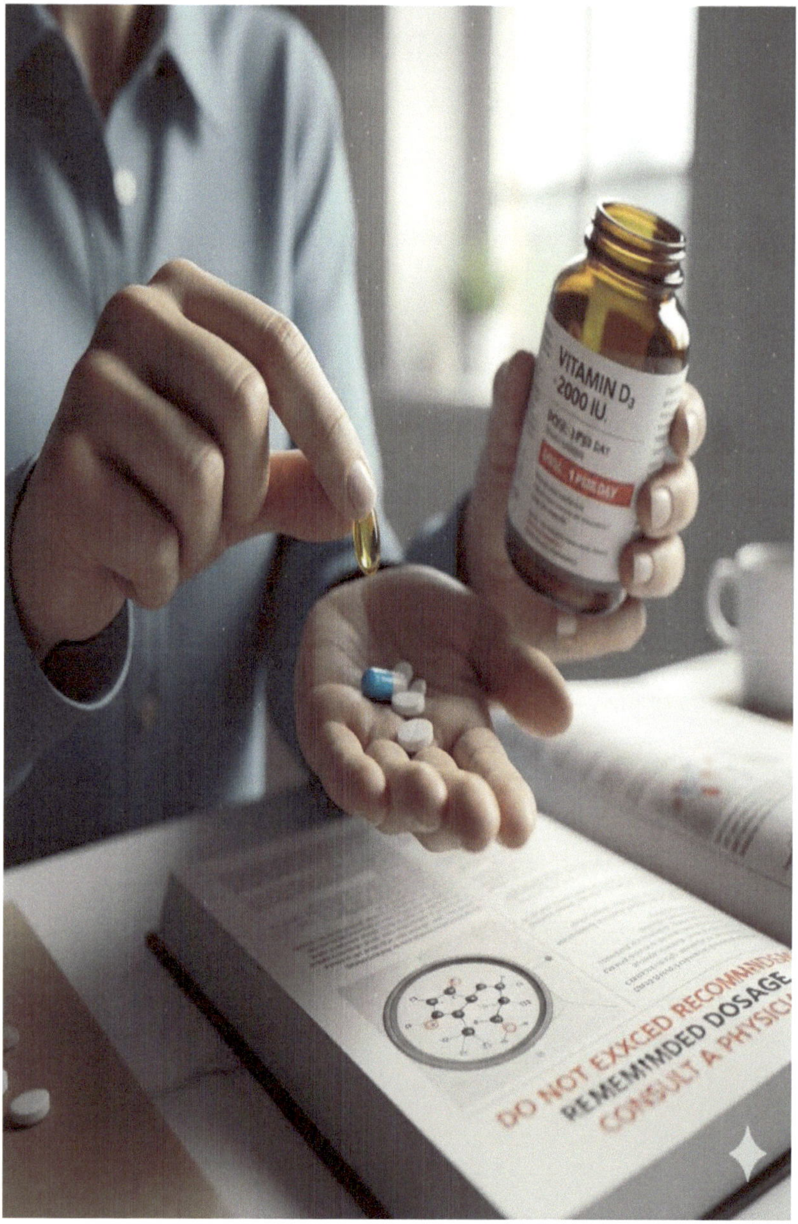
VITAMIN D3
2000 IU.
DO NOT EXXCED
REMEMMDED DOSAGE
CONSULT A

Too Much

1. Know the Difference Between Fat-Soluble and Water-Soluble Vitamins

- **Fat-soluble vitamins** (A, D, E, K) are stored in the body and can accumulate to toxic levels if taken in excess.
- **Water-soluble vitamins** (B-complex and C) are flushed out more easily, but extremely high doses can still cause problems such as nerve damage (B6), nausea, or digestive issues.

Understanding this helps you avoid unnecessary or excessive supplementation.

---

2. Follow Recommended Daily Allowances (RDAs)

Each vitamin has a safe limit. More is **not** better.

Exceeding the upper limit—especially for D, A, B6, E, or K—can lead to serious health issues such as organ damage, nerve problems, or bleeding disorders.

Always check dosage labels to ensure you stay within safe guidelines.

---

3. Avoid Taking Multiple Supplements With Overlapping Vitamins

Many supplements contain the same vitamins. For example:

- A multivitamin
- A hair/skin/nail supplement
- An energy booster
- A vitamin D capsule

Taking these together can unintentionally double or triple your dosage.

Read labels carefully to avoid stacking the same vitamins from multiple products.

---

4. Choose High-Quality Supplements With Clear Ingredient Labels

Cheap or poorly regulated supplements may contain higher doses than listed or include hidden ingredients. To stay safe:

- Choose products that are **third-party tested**
- Select reputable brands
- Avoid supplements with extremely high doses unless medically advised

Transparency in labeling is essential for preventing accidental overdose.

---

5. Consider Your Diet Before Adding Supplements

If you already consume fortified foods—like cereals, plant milks, protein shakes, or energy drinks—you may already be getting large amounts of certain vitamins.

Track how much you are receiving from both food and supplements combined.

---

6. Be Cautious With “Mega-Dose” or “High-Potency” Supplements

These products often contain far higher doses than your body needs. Unless recommended by a healthcare provider:

- Avoid mega doses of vitamins A, D, E, and K
- Avoid high-dose B6 supplements (may cause nerve damage)
- Use vitamin C and niacin in moderation

High potency does not mean high benefit.

---

7. Consider Medication Interactions

Some vitamins interact with prescription medications:

- Vitamin K affects blood thinners
- Vitamin D and calcium can interact with heart medications
- Vitamin A and isotretinoin together can be toxic

Always discuss supplements with a doctor if you are taking any medications.

---

8. Get Blood Tests When Needed

Regular testing helps identify which vitamins you truly need. Many adults take supplements they don't require, while missing the ones they actually lack.

Blood tests can prevent unnecessary or excessive supplementation.

---

9. Start Low and Increase Only if Necessary

When starting a new supplement, begin with the lowest effective dose.

Increase only if:

- A healthcare provider recommends it
- Blood tests show deficiency
- Symptoms or conditions justify higher intake

Slow, controlled adjustments reduce the risk of overdose.

---

10. Store Vitamins Safely and Use Properly

- Keep vitamins in labeled containers
- Avoid mixing pills from different bottles
- Follow daily dosage instructions carefully
- Never use expired supplements

Safe handling helps avoid accidental misuse.

Final Note

Vitamins are vital for health, but they must be taken mindfully. A balanced diet, a well-chosen supplement plan, and professional guidance help you get all the benefits of vitamins—without the risks of overdose. By being informed and cautious, you can protect your health while optimizing your nutrition.

Wrapping Up

Taking vitamin supplements simply because "everyone else is doing it" is not a good enough reason to begin a supplement routine. Likewise, adding vitamins without considering your overall lifestyle, diet, and health needs can do more harm than good.

For some people, supplements are used as a substitute for proper meals – a choice that can lead to nutritional imbalances. Vitamins are meant to **support**, not replace, a healthy diet. When taken without proper guidance, two outcomes often occur:

- The body may not absorb the vitamins efficiently, leading to a harmful buildup and potential medical complications.
- The body may simply flush out the excess, resulting in wasted money and no real health benefit.

Understanding how vitamins work, choosing them wisely, and using them responsibly are key to improving your overall health.

I hope this guide has given you a clearer and more confident understanding of vitamins and how they contribute to a healthier, more balanced lifestyle. If you make informed choices and listen to your body, you're already on the right path.

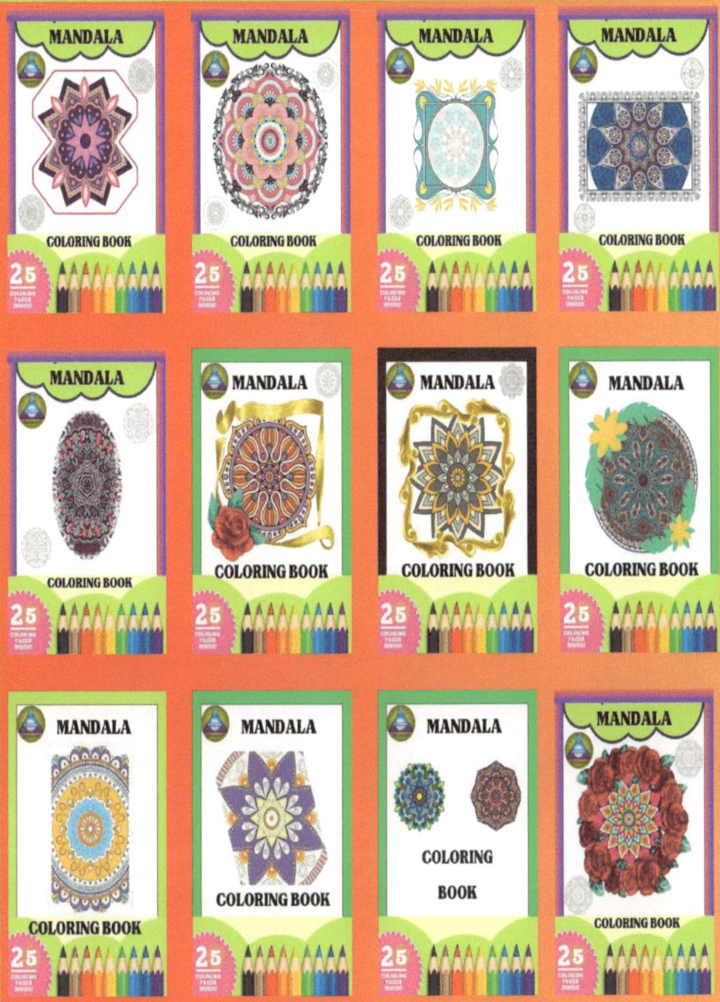

PUBLISHED BY THE BLJ KTS SERVICES.

Contact Us:

Gmail:bljktsservices@gmail.com

Phone No: 7351805039

ISBN No : 978-81-995902-3-6

www.ingramcontent.com/pod-product-compliance
Ingram Content Group UK Ltd.
Pitfield, Milton Keynes, MK11 3LW, UK
UKHW061433190726
13845UKWH00020B/165